HERBAL SOLUTIONS FOR PSORIASIS

A Comprehensive Guide for healing psoriasis

Dr Philip Ortner

Copyright © [2023] by [Dr Philip Ortner]

All rights reserved.

No part of this publication may be reproduced,

Distributed, or transmitted in any form or by any means, including

photocopying, recording, or other electronic or Mechanical

methods,

Without the prior written

Permission of the publisher

Except in the case of brief quotations embodied in critical reviews

and certain other

Publish by Dr Philip Ortner

Disclaimer: the opinion and views expressed in this book are
those of the author and do not necessarily reflect the policy or
position of any character or organization mention in this book

TABLE OF CONTENTS

CHAPTER 1

Introduction to Psoriasis

Psoriasis is more than just a skin condition; it's a chronic autoimmune disease that affects millions of people worldwide. To understand psoriasis, we need to delve into its definition, different types, how it manifests, its prevalence, and the significant impact it can have on individuals' lives. Additionally, we'll touch upon conventional treatments and their limitations, setting the stage for exploring alternative approaches, particularly the use of herbs.

Definition and Overview of Psoriasis

Psoriasis is a chronic skin disorder characterized by the rapid buildup of skin cells, leading to the formation of thick, silvery scales and red, inflamed patches. While it primarily affects the skin, it is crucial to recognize it as an autoimmune condition, meaning that the immune system mistakenly attacks healthy cells, causing an overproduction of skin cells. This process results in the characteristic symptoms of psoriasis, including itching, pain, and visible skin changes.

Understanding psoriasis goes beyond its external manifestations. It involves recognizing the intricate interplay between the immune system, genetic factors, and environmental triggers that contribute to its development. The immune system plays a central role in psoriasis, as it triggers an inflammatory response that accelerates the turnover of skin cells, leading to the formation of plaques.

Types and Manifestations of Psoriasis

Psoriasis comes in various forms, each with its own distinct characteristics. The most common type is plaque psoriasis, which presents as raised, red patches covered with a silvery-white buildup of dead skin cells. Other types include guttate psoriasis, characterized by small, dot-like lesions; inverse psoriasis, affecting skin folds; pustular psoriasis, featuring pus-filled blisters; and erythrodermic psoriasis, a severe and potentially life-threatening form that causes widespread redness and scaling.

The manifestations of psoriasis extend beyond the physical symptoms. The condition can impact an individual's emotional well-being, leading to feelings of self-consciousness, embarrassment, and even depression. The visible nature of psoriasis can make social interactions challenging, as individuals may face judgment or misunderstanding from others. Therefore, addressing the emotional and psychological aspects of psoriasis is an integral part of its management.

Prevalence and Impact on Individuals' Lives

Psoriasis is a prevalent condition, affecting people of all ages and ethnicities. The World Health Organization estimates that over 125 million people worldwide live with psoriasis. It is essential to highlight that psoriasis is not merely a cosmetic issue; it significantly influences the quality of life for those affected.

The impact of psoriasis extends beyond the physical discomfort and visible symptoms. Individuals with psoriasis may experience limitations in their daily activities, such as difficulty sleeping due to itching, challenges in maintaining personal relationships, and hindrances in pursuing certain occupations. The emotional toll can be substantial, with many individuals reporting feelings of isolation, low self-esteem, and a diminished sense of well-being.

Understanding the prevalence and impact of psoriasis emphasizes the need for comprehensive and compassionate approaches to its management. It is not only about treating the visible symptoms but also addressing the emotional and social aspects that contribute to the overall burden of the condition on individuals' lives.

Conventional Treatments and Their Limitations

While medical science has made significant strides in developing treatments for psoriasis, conventional approaches are not without limitations. Common treatments include topical corticosteroids, phototherapy, oral medications, and biologic drugs. These treatments aim to alleviate symptoms, reduce inflammation, and slow down the excessive skin cell turnover.

However, these treatments may not be universally effective, and individuals often face challenges such as the need for ongoing medication, potential side effects, and the financial burden of long-term treatment. Moreover, some individuals may not respond adequately to conventional therapies, prompting the exploration of alternative and complementary approaches.

In the pursuit of a more holistic and personalized approach to psoriasis management, individuals are increasingly turning to herbal solutions. Herbs offer the potential for addressing the root causes of psoriasis, reducing inflammation, and promoting overall skin health. This book will explore the diverse world of medicinal herbs, their therapeutic properties, and practical ways to incorporate them into a comprehensive psoriasis management plan.

CHAPTER 2

Understanding the Root Causes of Psoriasis

To truly comprehend psoriasis and explore effective ways to manage it, we must unravel the intricate web of factors that contribute to its development. Chapter 2 delves into the fundamental aspects that underlie psoriasis, providing insights into genetic predisposition, immune system dysfunction, environmental triggers, and the pivotal role of inflammation in this chronic condition.

Genetic Factors and Predisposition

One of the key components in understanding psoriasis lies within our genes. Genetic factors play a significant role in determining whether an individual is predisposed to developing psoriasis. If there's a family history of psoriasis, the likelihood of inheriting the genetic predisposition increases. However, having a genetic predisposition doesn't guarantee that an individual will develop psoriasis, as environmental factors also come into play.

Genes associated with psoriasis influence the immune system's response and the regeneration of skin cells. Certain variations in these genes can contribute to an overactive immune response and an accelerated production of skin cells, leading to the characteristic symptoms of psoriasis. While genetics lay the foundation, it's the interaction between genetic factors and environmental triggers that often determines whether psoriasis manifests.

Immune System Dysfunction

The immune system, our body's defense mechanism against invaders, plays a central role in psoriasis. In individuals with psoriasis, the immune system goes awry, mistakenly identifying healthy skin cells as foreign threats and launching an attack. This misguided immune response triggers inflammation and accelerates the turnover of skin cells, resulting in the formation of plaques.

A specific type of immune cell called T cells becomes overactive in psoriasis. These T cells, normally responsible for defending the body against infections, start attacking healthy skin cells. This immune dysfunction is a critical factor in the development and persistence of psoriasis. Understanding the immune system's role sheds light on why psoriasis is classified as an autoimmune disease.

Environmental Triggers

While genetics and immune system dysfunction set the stage for psoriasis, environmental triggers act as catalysts that can initiate or exacerbate the condition. Various environmental factors can contribute to the onset or flare-ups of psoriasis.

Common triggers include infections, particularly streptococcal infections, which can stimulate the immune system and worsen psoriasis symptoms.

Stress is another significant environmental trigger. High levels of stress can impact the immune system and exacerbate inflammation, potentially leading to psoriasis flare-ups. Lifestyle factors such as smoking and excessive alcohol consumption have also been linked to an increased risk of developing psoriasis or experiencing more severe symptoms.

Certain medications, such as lithium and beta-blockers, may trigger or worsen psoriasis in susceptible individuals. Additionally, physical trauma to the skin, known as the Koebner phenomenon, can cause psoriasis lesions to develop at the site of injury. Understanding these environmental triggers empowers individuals with psoriasis to make informed lifestyle choices and manage factors that may contribute to their condition.

The Role of Inflammation in Psoriasis

Inflammation is a natural and necessary response of the immune system to protect the body from injury and infection. However, in psoriasis, inflammation becomes chronic and misguided, leading to the hallmark symptoms of the condition. The inflammatory response in psoriasis primarily targets the skin, resulting in redness, swelling, and the formation of plaques.

Inflammatory cytokines, signaling molecules produced by immune cells, play a crucial role in orchestrating the inflammatory response in psoriasis. These cytokines contribute to the accelerated turnover of skin cells and the recruitment of immune cells to the affected areas. As a result, the skin cells don't have sufficient time to mature and slough off, leading to the accumulation of thickened, scaly skin.

Understanding the role of inflammation in psoriasis is pivotal in developing targeted treatments. Many conventional and emerging therapies aim to modulate the inflammatory response, either by suppressing specific immune activities or by interfering with the action of inflammatory cytokines. This knowledge also underscores the potential of anti-inflammatory herbs, a topic that will be explored in later chapters, in managing psoriasis symptoms by addressing the root cause of chronic inflammation.

CHAPTER 3

Herbs and Their Therapeutic Properties

Embarking on the journey of managing psoriasis with herbs requires a foundational understanding of medicinal herbs and their diverse therapeutic properties. In this chapter, we will explore the rich world of herbs, categorizing them based on their potential benefits for individuals grappling with psoriasis. From anti-inflammatory and immune-modulating herbs to those with skin-healing and detoxifying properties, this chapter serves as a guide to harnessing the healing potential of nature.

Overview of Medicinal Herbs

Medicinal herbs have been integral to traditional medicine systems for centuries, offering a natural and holistic approach to health. These plants contain a myriad of bioactive compounds, each with its unique properties that can positively impact the human body. From leaves and roots to flowers and seeds, different parts of these herbs are used to create remedies that address various health concerns.

The use of medicinal herbs for managing psoriasis is rooted in their ability to target the underlying factors contributing to the condition, such as inflammation, immune dysfunction, and impaired skin healing. Understanding the diverse range of herbs and their therapeutic properties empowers individuals to tailor their approach to psoriasis management, embracing a holistic and personalized strategy.

Anti-Inflammatory Herbs

Chronic inflammation lies at the heart of psoriasis, driving the symptoms and perpetuating the cycle of skin cell overgrowth. Anti-inflammatory herbs, with their natural ability to dampen excessive inflammation, emerge as valuable allies in the quest for psoriasis management.

Turmeric is a standout anti-inflammatory herb, thanks to its active compound curcumin. Curcumin has demonstrated potent anti-inflammatory effects, inhibiting specific molecules that play a role in the inflammatory cascade. Incorporating turmeric into one's diet or using it topically may help alleviate redness and swelling associated with psoriasis lesions.

Ginger is another herb with notable anti-inflammatory properties. It contains gingerol, a bioactive compound that has been shown to reduce inflammation and modulate the immune response. Whether consumed as a tea or used topically, ginger can be a soothing addition to a psoriasis management routine.

Immune-Modulating Herbs

Given the autoimmune nature of psoriasis, herbs with immune-modulating properties can help rebalance the immune system and curb its overactive response.

Echinacea is a well-known immune-modulating herb that has been traditionally used to support the immune system. By regulating immune responses, echinacea may help modulate the inflammatory processes involved in psoriasis. Whether consumed as a tea or in supplement form, echinacea is considered a gentle yet effective herb for immune support.

Astragalus is another immune-modulating herb that has been valued in traditional Chinese medicine. It is believed to strengthen the immune system while promoting balance. Incorporating astragalus into a psoriasis management plan may help address the underlying immune dysfunction associated with the condition.

Skin-Healing Herbs

Psoriasis not only involves inflammation and immune dysfunction but also impaired skin healing. Herbs with skin-healing properties can aid in the restoration of damaged skin, promoting a healthier and more resilient epidermis.

Calendula, also known as marigold, is a renowned skin-healing herb. It possesses anti-inflammatory and antimicrobial properties, making it a valuable addition to topical preparations. Calendula can help soothe irritated skin and promote the healing of psoriasis lesions.

Lavender is not only prized for its aromatic qualities but also for its skin-healing properties. Lavender essential oil, when diluted and applied topically, may contribute to the healing process and reduce skin irritation associated with psoriasis.

Detoxifying Herbs

Toxins in the body can contribute to the inflammatory processes seen in psoriasis. Detoxifying herbs assist the body in eliminating these toxins, promoting overall health and potentially alleviating psoriasis symptoms.

Dandelion is a well-known detoxifying herb that supports liver function, the body's primary detox organ. By aiding the liver in processing and eliminating toxins, dandelion may contribute to a reduction in inflammatory responses. Whether consumed as a tea or as part of a salad, dandelion is a versatile herb with detoxifying benefits.

Milk thistle is another herb celebrated for its detoxifying properties, particularly in supporting liver health. The active compound silymarin in milk thistle has antioxidant and anti-inflammatory effects, making it a valuable herb in the context of psoriasis management.

In conclusion, Chapter 3 provides a comprehensive exploration of medicinal herbs and their therapeutic properties, categorizing them based on their potential benefits for individuals dealing with psoriasis. From anti-inflammatory and immune-modulating herbs to those with skin-healing and detoxifying properties, these herbs offer a holistic approach to addressing the root causes of psoriasis. As readers delve into the world of herbal solutions, they gain valuable insights into the diverse array of plants that nature provides, each offering a unique contribution to the journey of psoriasis management. Armed with this knowledge, individuals can make informed choices about incorporating herbs into their lifestyle, embracing a personalized and holistic approach to managing this chronic condition.

CHAPTER 4

Herbal Approaches to Managing Psoriasis Symptoms

Managing the symptoms of psoriasis involves addressing a spectrum of challenges, from the persistent itching and irritation to the visible redness and inflammation of the skin. Chapter 4 delves into herbal solutions that offer relief across various dimensions of psoriasis symptoms. This chapter guides readers through the practical application of herbs in alleviating discomfort, reducing inflammation, promoting skin hydration, slowing down skin cell overgrowth, and addressing associated conditions, such as arthritis.

Alleviating Itching and Irritation

Itching and irritation are among the most pervasive and distressing symptoms of psoriasis. Herbal remedies can offer soothing relief, providing comfort to individuals navigating the often relentless urge to scratch.

Aloe Vera stands out as a natural remedy for alleviating itching and irritation. The gel extracted from the leaves of the aloe vera plant has cooling and anti-inflammatory properties. Applying aloe vera gel to psoriasis-affected areas can provide immediate relief, helping to soothe the skin and reduce itching.

Chamomile is another herb renowned for its calming effects. Whether used as a topical ointment or in the form of a chamomile tea compress, this herb can help ease itching and irritation. Chamomile's anti-inflammatory and skin-soothing properties make it a valuable ally in the daily management of psoriasis symptoms.

Reducing Redness and Inflammation

The characteristic redness and inflammation associated with psoriasis are manifestations of the underlying inflammatory processes. Herbal remedies with anti-inflammatory properties can help mitigate these symptoms, promoting a more comfortable and visually soothing experience.

Calendula, with its anti-inflammatory properties, can be applied topically to reduce redness and inflammation. Calendula-infused creams or ointments can be gently massaged onto affected areas, offering relief and contributing to the overall healing of psoriasis lesions.

Licorice Root contains compounds that exhibit anti-inflammatory effects. Applying licorice root extract topically may help reduce redness and inflammation associated with psoriasis. It's important to note that licorice root should be used cautiously, and consulting with a healthcare professional is advised.

Promoting Skin Hydration

Psoriasis often leads to dry, flaky skin, exacerbating discomfort and contributing to the persistence of symptoms. Herbal solutions that promote skin hydration can play a crucial role in managing psoriasis symptoms.

Coconut Oil is a versatile herbal remedy known for its moisturizing properties. Applying coconut oil to psoriasis-affected areas can help alleviate dryness and reduce scaling. The oil forms a protective layer on the skin, preventing moisture loss and promoting hydration.

Oatmeal is not only a soothing addition to the bath but also a herbal remedy for promoting skin hydration. Oatmeal baths can provide relief from itching and help moisturize the skin. The gentle, hydrating properties of oatmeal make it a suitable option for individuals with psoriasis.

Slowing Down Skin Cell Overgrowth

One of the core challenges in psoriasis is the accelerated turnover of skin cells, leading to the formation of plaques. Herbal remedies that can help regulate skin cell growth play a vital role in managing this aspect of psoriasis.

Oregon Grape is an herb with properties that may inhibit the abnormal growth of skin cells. Compounds in Oregon grape, such as berberine, have been studied for their potential in slowing down the proliferation of skin cells. This herb can be incorporated into topical preparations or used as part of an herbal regimen for psoriasis management.

Neem is another herb that has been traditionally used for its anti-proliferative properties. Applying neem oil or neem-based creams to psoriasis lesions may help regulate the growth of skin cells. Neem's antibacterial and anti-inflammatory effects further contribute to its potential in managing psoriasis symptoms.

Addressing Associated Conditions (e.g., Arthritis)

Psoriasis is not confined to the skin; it can also manifest as psoriatic arthritis, a condition that affects the joints. Herbal remedies that address associated conditions, such as arthritis, offer a holistic approach to managing the diverse manifestations of psoriasis.

Turmeric emerges once again as a potent herbal remedy, this time for managing arthritis symptoms associated with psoriatic arthritis. Curcumin, the active compound in turmeric, exhibits anti-inflammatory and analgesic properties that may help alleviate joint pain and stiffness. Incorporating turmeric into the diet or taking it as a supplement can contribute to overall joint health.

Ginger is another herb known for its anti-inflammatory effects, making it a valuable addition to the arsenal against arthritis symptoms. Whether consumed as a tea or included in meals, ginger can help individuals with psoriatic arthritis manage joint pain and improve mobility.

CHAPTER 5

Building a Psoriasis-Friendly Diet with Herbs

Diet plays a pivotal role in managing psoriasis, influencing inflammation, immune function, and overall skin health. Chapter 5 guides readers through the impact of diet on psoriasis, highlighting anti-inflammatory food choices, the incorporation of herbs as culinary additives, the benefits of herbal teas, and the creation of psoriasis-friendly recipes. By understanding the relationship between diet and psoriasis, individuals can empower themselves to make informed choices that contribute to their overall well-being.

The Impact of Diet on Psoriasis

The old adage "you are what you eat" holds particular significance for individuals with psoriasis. While diet may not be a direct cause of psoriasis, certain food choices can either exacerbate or alleviate symptoms. Understanding the impact of diet on psoriasis involves recognizing the interplay between inflammation, immune response, and skin health.

Highly processed foods, sugary snacks, and excessive alcohol consumption can contribute to inflammation in the body, potentially triggering or worsening psoriasis symptoms. On the other hand, a diet rich in anti-inflammatory foods, nutrient-dense fruits and vegetables, and hydration can positively influence the body's response to psoriasis.

Anti-Inflammatory Food Choices

Anti-inflammatory foods form the cornerstone of a psoriasis-friendly dict. These foods help modulate the immune response, reduce inflammation, and support overall health. Herbs, with their potent anti-inflammatory properties, can be valuable additions to meals.

Turmeric stands out as a potent anti-inflammatory herb, thanks to its active compound curcumin. Incorporating turmeric into meals, either by sprinkling it on vegetables or adding it to sauces, can contribute to the overall anti-inflammatory profile of the diet.

Ginger is another herb with anti-inflammatory properties. Whether used in stir-fries, grated into salads, or brewed into a soothing tea, ginger can enhance the anti-inflammatory potential of meals.

Herbs as Culinary Additives

Herbs aren't just flavor enhancers; they also bring a host of health benefits to the table. Integrating herbs as culinary additives can elevate the nutritional content of meals while providing a burst of natural flavors.

Rosemary, for example, not only adds a delightful aroma to dishes but also brings anti-inflammatory and antioxidant properties to the table. Roasting vegetables with a sprinkle of rosemary or infusing olive oil with this herb can be a delicious way to incorporate its benefits into meals.

Basil, with its fresh and aromatic profile, is a versatile herb that pairs well with salads, pasta, and various dishes. Beyond its culinary appeal, basil contains compounds that exhibit anti-inflammatory and antimicrobial effects, contributing to both flavor and health.

Herbal Teas and Their Benefits

Herbal teas offer a comforting and hydrating way to incorporate the benefits of herbs into a psoriasis-friendly diet. Beyond hydration, certain herbal teas boast properties that can positively impact inflammation and promote overall well-being.

Chamomile Tea is not only renowned for its calming effects but also for its anti-inflammatory properties. Sipping on chamomile tea can provide a soothing experience, potentially contributing to the management of psoriasis symptoms.

Green Tea is rich in antioxidants, particularly catechins, which have anti-inflammatory and immune-modulating effects. Regular consumption of green tea can be a healthful addition to a psoriasis-friendly diet, offering hydration and potential benefits for skin health.

Recipes for Psoriasis-Friendly Meals

Creating psoriasis-friendly meals involves a thoughtful selection of ingredients that align with an anti-inflammatory and nutrient-dense approach. Here are a few recipe ideas that incorporate herbs and support a diet conducive to managing psoriasis:

- **Turmeric-Spiced Vegetable Stir-Fry:**

- Ingredients: Mixed vegetables (bell peppers, broccoli, carrots), tofu or chicken, turmeric, ginger, garlic, soy sauce.
  - Method: Sauté vegetables and protein in a pan with turmeric, ginger, and garlic. Finish with a splash of soy sauce for flavor.

- **Mediterranean Herb-Roasted Salmon:**
  - Ingredients: Salmon fillets, rosemary, thyme, oregano, lemon, olive oil, salt, and pepper.
  - Method: Marinate salmon with herbs, olive oil, lemon juice, salt, and pepper. Roast in the oven until cooked through.

- **Basil Pesto Zucchini Noodles:**
  - Ingredients: Zucchini noodles, cherry tomatoes, pine nuts, basil, garlic, Parmesan cheese, olive oil.

o Method: Make a pesto sauce with basil, garlic, pine nuts, Parmesan, and olive oil. Toss with zucchini noodles and cherry tomatoes.

These recipes showcase how herbs can be seamlessly integrated into meals, adding both flavor and health benefits. The emphasis is on whole, nutrient-dense ingredients that align with an anti-inflammatory approach, promoting a diet conducive to managing psoriasis symptoms.

CHAPTER 6

Integrating Herbs into Your Daily Routine

Managing psoriasis involves more than just dietary changes; it's about incorporating herbs into your daily routine to address symptoms and promote overall skin health. Chapter 6 guides readers through practical ways to seamlessly integrate herbs into their daily lives. From creating herbal skincare products to incorporating herbs into bath routines, using herbal compresses and poultices, and exploring herbal supplements, this chapter provides a holistic approach to making herbs a natural and beneficial part of everyday life.

Creating Herbal Skincare Products

Skincare is a crucial aspect of managing psoriasis, and herbs can play a significant role in creating soothing and nourishing products. Herbal skincare products offer a gentle and natural approach to caring for psoriasis-affected skin.

Calendula-infused Oil is a simple yet effective way to harness the healing properties of calendula for skincare. Calendula, with its anti-inflammatory and skin-soothing qualities, can be infused into carrier oils like jojoba or almond oil. This infused oil can be applied topically to psoriasis lesions to help reduce redness and inflammation.

Aloe Vera Gel with Lavender: Combine the cooling and moisturizing properties of aloe vera with the soothing effects of lavender essential oil. Mix aloe vera gel with a few drops of lavender oil and apply it to affected areas. This blend can provide relief from itching and irritation associated with psoriasis.

Incorporating Herbs into Bath Routines

Baths can be a therapeutic and relaxing part of a psoriasis management routine. Adding herbs to baths can enhance their healing benefits, providing relief for both the skin and the mind.

Oatmeal Bath Soak: Oatmeal has soothing properties that can benefit irritated skin. Simply grind oats into a fine powder and add it to warm bathwater. Soaking in an oatmeal bath can help alleviate itching and promote skin hydration.

Lavender and Chamomile Bath Salts: Combine Epsom salts with dried lavender and chamomile flowers to create fragrant and soothing bath salts. The calming aroma of lavender and chamomile, coupled with the muscle-relaxing properties of Epsom salts, can make bath time a therapeutic experience.

Herbal Compresses and Poultices

Herbal compresses and poultices offer localized relief for psoriasis-affected areas. These applications can be particularly beneficial for reducing inflammation and promoting healing.

Comfrey Compress: Comfrey is known for its skin-healing properties. Create a compress by steeping dried comfrey leaves in hot water, allowing the mixture to cool slightly, and then applying it to psoriasis lesions. Comfrey can aid in reducing inflammation and supporting the healing process.

Turmeric Poultice: Harness the anti-inflammatory power of turmeric by creating a poultice. Mix turmeric powder with water to create a paste and apply it to psoriasis-affected areas. Leave it on for a short period before rinsing off. This turmeric poultice can help alleviate redness and inflammation.

Herbal Supplements and Their Proper Use

In addition to incorporating herbs topically, herbal supplements can complement a holistic approach to psoriasis management. However, it's crucial to use them with care and under the guidance of healthcare professionals.

Evening Primrose Oil: Evening primrose oil, rich in gamma-linolenic acid (GLA), is believed to have anti-inflammatory properties. Taking evening primrose oil supplements may help modulate inflammation associated with psoriasis. Consult with a healthcare provider for appropriate dosage and usage.

Milk Thistle Supplements: Milk thistle is known for its detoxifying effects on the liver. As the liver plays a role in processing toxins that can contribute to inflammation, milk thistle supplements may support overall liver health. However, it's important to use them cautiously and under professional guidance.

Summary: Chapter 6 encourages individuals to weave herbs into their daily routines, transforming them from mere remedies to integral elements of self-care. From creating herbal skincare products that cater to the specific needs of psoriasis-affected skin to incorporating herbs into bath routines for therapeutic relaxation, using herbal compresses and poultices for localized relief, and exploring herbal supplements for internal support, this chapter provides a diverse set of tools for individuals on their psoriasis management journey.

The integration of herbs into daily life is not only practical but also empowers individuals to take an active role in their well-being. The calming effects of herbal bath rituals, the targeted relief of compresses and poultices, and the internal support of herbal supplements collectively contribute to a comprehensive and personalized approach to managing psoriasis.

However, it's crucial to approach the use of herbs with mindfulness and consult with healthcare professionals, especially when considering herbal supplements. While herbs offer valuable natural support, they should complement, not replace, conventional medical advice and treatments. By blending the wisdom of traditional herbal remedies with modern healthcare guidance, individuals can create a daily routine that nurtures both their skin and overall health.

CHAPTER 7

Case Studies and Success Stories

In the journey of managing psoriasis, the experiences of others who have walked a similar path can be a beacon of hope and guidance. Chapter 7 delves into personal accounts of individuals who successfully managed their psoriasis with the help of herbs. By exploring different approaches, combinations that worked, lessons learned from successful cases, and offering encouragement for readers to discover what works best for them, this chapter aims to inspire and empower those seeking effective and holistic solutions for psoriasis.

Personal Accounts of Individuals Managing Psoriasis with Herbs

The power of personal narratives lies in their ability to resonate and connect with others facing similar challenges. In this chapter, individuals share their stories of navigating the complexities of psoriasis and finding relief through herbal approaches.

Sarah's Journey with Turmeric and Aloe Vera: Sarah, a 32-year-old teacher, struggled with persistent psoriasis flare-ups. Frustrated with the limitations of conventional treatments, she turned to herbal remedies. Sarah found relief by incorporating turmeric supplements into her daily routine, harnessing the anti-inflammatory benefits of curcumin. Additionally, she applied aloe vera gel topically, experiencing soothing effects that alleviated itching and redness. Sarah's journey showcases the potential of combining internal and external herbal approaches for managing psoriasis.

Mark's Success with Dietary Changes and Herbal Teas: Mark, a 45-year-old IT professional, noticed a correlation between his diet and psoriasis symptoms. By adopting a psoriasis-friendly diet rich in anti-inflammatory foods, Mark experienced a noticeable reduction in redness and inflammation. He complemented dietary changes with herbal teas, particularly chamomile and green tea, which contributed to his overall well-being. Mark's case highlights the impact of lifestyle and dietary modifications, demonstrating that holistic changes can yield positive results.

Different Approaches and Combinations that Worked

Psoriasis is a diverse condition, and what works for one person may not necessarily work for another. This chapter explores the varied approaches and combinations that individuals have found effective in managing their psoriasis symptoms.

Emily's Herbal Skincare Routine: Emily, a 28-year-old graphic designer, developed a personalized herbal skincare routine to address her psoriasis-affected skin. She crafted a soothing salve using herbs like calendula, lavender, and chamomile infused into coconut oil. Emily's topical application provided her with relief from itching and contributed to the healing of psoriasis lesions. Her case underscores the importance of tailoring herbal approaches to individual preferences and needs.

James' Comprehensive Herbal Regimen: James, a 38-year-old fitness instructor, embraced a comprehensive herbal regimen that included dietary changes, herbal supplements, and topical applications. He incorporated turmeric and ginger into his meals, took evening primrose oil supplements, and applied a herbal ointment containing neem and aloe vera. James's multifaceted approach illustrates the potential benefits of combining various herbs to address different aspects of psoriasis.

Lessons Learned from Successful Cases

Examining successful cases provides valuable insights into the lessons learned on the path to managing psoriasis with herbs.

Consistency is Key: Many success stories emphasize the importance of consistency in applying herbal remedies. Whether it's taking herbal supplements daily, maintaining a psoriasis-friendly diet, or using herbal skincare products regularly, a consistent approach appears to yield more sustained results.

Personalization Matters: The diversity of approaches underscores the significance of personalized strategies. What works for one person may not work for another, emphasizing the need for individuals to explore and discover the herbal combinations and routines that align with their unique circumstances.

Holistic Approaches Show Promise: Successful cases often involve a holistic approach that addresses various facets of psoriasis, including dietary changes, herbal supplements, topical applications, and lifestyle modifications. This holistic perspective reflects the interconnected nature of health and encourages individuals to consider a comprehensive approach.

Encouragement for Readers to Explore What Works Best for Them

The chapter concludes by encouraging readers to embark on their unique journey of exploration, emphasizing that managing psoriasis is a personalized endeavor. While the case studies provide inspiration and insights, readers are reminded that their experience may differ, and it's essential to be open to discovering what works best for them.

Embrace a Trial-and-Error Mindset: Managing psoriasis with herbs is not a one-size-fits-all endeavor. Readers are encouraged to approach their journey with a trial-and-error mindset, understanding that finding the most effective herbal solutions may require some experimentation.

Consult with Healthcare Professionals: Seeking guidance from healthcare professionals is crucial throughout the process. Whether exploring herbal supplements or making significant lifestyle changes, consulting with healthcare providers ensures that individuals receive personalized advice and monitoring.

Celebrate Small Wins: The path to managing psoriasis can be challenging, but celebrating small wins along the way is vital. Each positive change, no matter how incremental, contributes to the overall well-being of individuals dealing with psoriasis.

CHAPTER 8

Lifestyle Changes for Long-Term Psoriasis Management

Beyond herbs and topical treatments, lifestyle changes play a crucial role in long-term psoriasis management. Chapter 8 delves into practical and impactful adjustments that individuals can make to foster overall well-being and alleviate psoriasis symptoms. This chapter explores stress management techniques, the importance of regular exercise, the impact of sleep hygiene on psoriasis, the role of mind-body practices like yoga and meditation, and encourages readers to embrace a holistic approach to health.

Stress Management Techniques

Stress is a known trigger for psoriasis flare-ups, making stress management a key component of long-term management. This section explores practical techniques to mitigate stress and promote emotional well-being.

Deep Breathing Exercises: Simple yet effective, deep breathing exercises can help activate the body's relaxation response. Taking slow, deep breaths and focusing on the breath can calm the nervous system, reducing stress levels. Deep breathing can be practiced anywhere, providing a quick and accessible stress-relief tool.

Mindfulness and Mindful Meditation: Mindfulness involves staying present in the moment without judgment. Mindful meditation, which often incorporates focused breathing and awareness exercises, can help individuals manage stress. Regular mindfulness practices contribute to a more balanced and resilient mindset.

Artistic Outlets: Engaging in creative activities, whether it's painting, writing, or playing a musical instrument, provides an outlet for self-expression and stress relief. These activities offer a break from the demands of daily life and foster a sense of accomplishment and joy.

The Importance of Regular Exercise

Exercise is not only beneficial for overall health but can also play a role in managing psoriasis. This section explores the impact of regular physical activity on psoriasis symptoms.

Aerobic Exercise: Activities like brisk walking, jogging, or cycling can promote cardiovascular health and contribute to stress reduction. The increased circulation associated with aerobic exercise may also have positive effects on skin health.

Strength Training: Building muscle through strength training exercises can enhance overall fitness and support joint health. Strong muscles can provide better support for joints affected by psoriatic arthritis, a condition that can accompany psoriasis.

Low-Impact Activities: For individuals with joint pain or mobility issues, low-impact activities like swimming or yoga can offer the benefits of exercise without excessive stress on joints. These activities promote flexibility and strength.

Sleep Hygiene and Its Impact on Psoriasis

Quality sleep is essential for overall health, and its impact on psoriasis should not be underestimated. This section explores the connection between sleep hygiene and psoriasis symptoms.

Consistent Sleep Schedule: Maintaining a regular sleep schedule, going to bed and waking up at the same time each day, helps regulate the body's internal clock. Consistent sleep patterns contribute to better sleep quality.

Create a Relaxing Bedtime Routine: Establishing a calming routine before bedtime signals to the body that it's time to wind down. This can include activities like reading a book, taking a warm bath, or practicing relaxation exercises.

Optimize Sleep Environment: Creating a comfortable sleep environment involves keeping the bedroom cool, dark, and quiet. Investing in a comfortable mattress and pillows can also improve sleep quality.

Mind-Body Practices (e.g., Yoga, Meditation)

The mind and body are intricately connected, and mind-body practices can positively impact both mental well-being and physical health. This section explores the benefits of incorporating practices like yoga and meditation into a psoriasis management routine.

Yoga: Yoga combines physical postures, breathwork, and meditation. The gentle stretching and strengthening exercises in yoga can improve flexibility and reduce stress. Certain yoga poses are specifically designed to benefit joint health, which can be particularly beneficial for individuals with psoriatic arthritis.

Meditation: Meditation involves cultivating mindfulness and a focused awareness. Regular meditation practice can help individuals manage stress, reduce anxiety, and promote a sense of calm. Meditation techniques can be tailored to suit individual preferences, making it accessible to a wide range of people.

Encouragement for a Holistic Approach to Health

This section emphasizes the importance of embracing a holistic approach to health that considers the interconnected nature of physical, mental, and emotional well-being.

Nutrition and Hydration: A balanced and nutrient-rich diet is essential for overall health and can contribute to psoriasis management. Adequate hydration is also crucial for skin health. Emphasizing whole foods, such as fruits, vegetables, and lean proteins, supports the body's nutritional needs.

Social Connections: Building and maintaining social connections can contribute to emotional well-being. Having a support system in place can provide encouragement, understanding, and shared experiences. Whether through friends, family, or support groups, social connections are a vital aspect of holistic health.

Regular Health Check-ups: While lifestyle changes play a significant role, regular check-ups with healthcare professionals are essential.

Monitoring overall health, addressing specific medical concerns, and staying informed about new developments in psoriasis management are crucial components of a holistic approach.

Summary: Chapter 8 underscores the significance of lifestyle changes for long-term psoriasis management. By incorporating stress management techniques, regular exercise, optimal sleep hygiene, and mind-body practices like yoga and meditation, individuals can foster a holistic approach to health that complements other aspects of psoriasis management, including herbal remedies and medical interventions.

The encouragement to embrace a holistic perspective is a reminder that managing psoriasis involves caring for the whole person—body, mind, and spirit. By actively participating in their well-being and making thoughtful lifestyle choices, individuals can contribute to the long-term management of psoriasis and improve their overall quality of life. The key is to approach these lifestyle changes with patience, consistency, and a commitment to personal well-being, understanding that each positive step is a valuable contribution to the journey of psoriasis management.

CONCLUSION

In conclusion, the exploration of herbs for psoriasis management has unfolded across eight informative chapters, each offering valuable insights and practical guidance. The journey begins with an introduction to psoriasis, providing a comprehensive understanding of the condition's definition, manifestations, prevalence, and the limitations of conventional treatments. Moving deeper, the root causes of psoriasis are explored, touching on genetic factors, immune system dysfunction, environmental triggers, and the role of inflammation.

The subsequent chapters guide readers through the therapeutic properties of medicinal herbs, herbal approaches to managing psoriasis symptoms, and the integration of herbs into dietary choices. From alleviating itching and inflammation to promoting skin hydration and regulating skin cell growth, herbs offer a multifaceted approach to psoriasis management. The importance of a psoriasis-friendly diet, enriched with anti-inflammatory herbs and herbal teas, is emphasized, providing a foundation for holistic well-being.

Beyond herbal remedies, lifestyle changes take center stage in Chapter 8, showcasing the interconnected nature of health and the integral role of stress management, regular exercise, sleep hygiene, and mind-body practices in long-term psoriasis management. The chapter encourages a holistic approach, emphasizing the significance of nutrition, social connections, and regular health check-ups in maintaining overall well-being.

The inclusion of case studies and success stories in Chapter 7 humanizes the psoriasis management journey, offering encouragement and practical lessons from those who have navigated the challenges successfully. These narratives underscore the importance of individualized approaches, consistency, and a willingness to explore what works best for each person.

Throughout the book, the underlying theme is empowerment—empowering individuals to take an active role in their psoriasis management journey. Whether through the use of herbs, dietary choices, lifestyle adjustments, or the wisdom shared in personal stories, the goal is to provide a holistic toolkit that addresses the diverse dimensions of psoriasis.